It's Never Too Late

You're Thinner Than You Think

By Louise N. Rotondo

DEDICATED TO MY MOTHER
MILDRED PERNA NAPPA

Published 2002
Revised 2013

Manufactured in the United States of America

1

INTRODUCTION

It is often said, you can never be too rich or too thin. As recent experience has shown, ways to get rich abound, but ways to get thin are hard to come by.

Louise, my wife for sixty-two years, has certainly proven that she has found the way to being thin and staying that way. Her expertise in the area of weight control is well evidenced by her own slim, healthy appearance, and zest for life as she happily enjoys her Golden Years.

Vincent J. Rotondo, Sr

TABLE OF CONTENTS

Chapter One
Introduction

Age is relative; it's only a number. Youth is but a fleeting glimpse of life and everything goes downhill after forty. Well, don't you believe it? I decided when I was forty that I wasn't going to let it happen to me and that I was going to keep what I had and I was going to improve upon it. Now more than thirty-two years later I believe I have succeeded.

At seventy-two years of age my body, my physical being and most gratifyingly my appearance is better now than when I was twenty-five. I have accomplished this modern day miracle with one simple thing, done before each meal, that I am going to share with you.

Having a youthful appearance is possible at any age providing you are able to allow the thin person you really are to come out and greet the world. That person really does exist inside yourself and by doing as I have done you will be able to show your true self to the world and be proud of who you really are. You will find you have a better attitude as you slim down and your physical appearance improves. Additionally, and even more important, you will feel better physically because you will become a healthier person in the process.

After the birth of my last child I weighed one hundred and fifty-five pounds and felt as though I couldn't get out of my own way. I was not happy with my weight which I believed to be about forty pounds more than it should have been for a person my height and age. I was even less happy with my appearance. I was obese. I resolved to do something about this and began to implement my plan. Within a few months my weight decreased and leveled off at about one-hundred and eight pounds where, give or take one or two pounds, it's remained ever since.

Accomplishing this did not require any strenuous efforts or even introducing any special exercises. It did not require the use of a personal trainer or dietician, or for that matter following any special diet what so ever, like the many professional models and other celebrities who struggle to keep their weight under control. During pre-retirement years most of us are busy working, raising children or doing both and can't afford to spend the time or money required to follow those types of special fitness regimen.

Think about the last wedding you went to and remember the beautiful, slim, radiant vision the bride was as she walked down the aisle and later graced the floor during the wedding dance with her new husband. Chances are you also knew her, as she no doubt was, several months before her wedding when she was a much heavier girl. Later most likely, you witnessed that modern day transformation right back to her former or even greater weight.

Well of course, it happens all the time, the bride wants to look her best on her wedding day and will subject herself to whatever it takes for the short time before the wedding to achieve the desired result. However, the short-term crash diet, usually a starvation one, is not something anyone can sustain, nor is it wise to do so. The results are unavoidable, but not if you do as I have done all these years having been able to effectively and simply control my weight and be satisfied with all that I eat at the same time.

After the wedding of course that beautiful vision that you saw walk down the aisle probably became a homemaker and career woman and in many cases a working mother. Now there's a recipe for self-neglect and natural tendency to gain weight for yielding to a heavy dependence on convenience foods. Certainly nowhere in that scenario would she find time for a physical fitness program, or for following the dictates of a diet counselor. No, during those times we really had more important things to concentrate on, or so we thought at the time, rather than the increased weight we never seemed to be able to get rid of.

Trying to stay on a specific diet is most often impossible due to the need to routinely cook for a family of hungry but choosy eaters. Keeping everyone satisfied usually means that your specific dietary plans and needs generally aren't met. All too often the busy homemaker resorts to going hungry, starving herself to lose the desired pounds.

This is usually followed by an eating binge to make up for the lost satisfaction of eating during the starvation period. What happens then, the weight is right back and maybe more than was taken off to begin with.

I'm sure you have noticed that this yo-yo routine with the weight coming on, going off and coming back on again, does a couple of things to your once young and tight body. Your skin starts to hang from being stretched like a rubber band. Well, even a rubber band gets stretch out of shape when it is repeatedly stretched even if it hasn't gone beyond its elastic limit. Your skin has an elastic limit like all materials do. Exceed it or simply stretch it too many times and it will sag and lose its nice tight youthful feel and appearance.

Additionally, after each dietary fling where you succeed in losing weight, the weight comes back quicker than it did during the previous cycle. Some people gain and lose weight so often that they have to resort to surgery to remove the hanging flesh.

Not even exercise is capable of tightening up the badly deformed, unsightly hanging skin.

Speaking of exercise, many people find out that this alone, while generally good for your cardiovascular system, is not sufficient to help you lose weight or even to maintain a desirable weight level. Exercising strenuously when you're overweight could be detrimental to your health and should not be viewed as a viable way of losing weight. You could lose more than the weight. The only way to get the weight off and reliably keep it off is to control your intake of food as I have been able to do for all these years by the simple expedient of drinking a proper amount of water in a timely way every day.

Ponce de Leon probably never realized how right he was when he was searching for the fountain of youth. He should have known he didn't have to travel across an ocean to find it, as it was available to him as it has been to anyone who has access to a decent supply of drinking water. It is available to you, all you need to do is tap into it and put it to work for you. Mother Nature will do the rest. In the next chapter I will describe in detail how to implement this regiment to get the best results and in the process let that thinner person who is the real you come out and show herself or himself to the world.

Chapter Two
HOW TO DO IT!

A long time ago, way back when your mother was imparting the wisdom of the ages to your youthful world of amazing discoveries, you might recall her telling you how important it was to drink at least eight glasses of water each day. Well, of course, like so many things our mother's told us, we've had to find a lot of them out for ourselves through our own experiences. Then, only to realize how easier it all would have been if only we had listened, and heeded the sagacious advice borne out by the experience of her lifetime.

I drink when I'm thirsty, you say, and that's the way most of us go about it, but there's more to it than that. Slaking a thirst might be rewarding experience at the time, but you would be far better off not having had the experience. Rather if you simply implemented the regimen that I am about to describe, you would benefit greatly by doing so and never have to worry about dehydration and its resulting craving to drink. The body after all is basically water with many other elements and compounds thrown into the soup of life, but the principal vehicle is the water in which all our bodily functions slosh around.

The bodies regulatory mechanisms do a miraculous job of keeping the chemistry of all its water based fluids in proper balance. Water replenishments to the systems are a fundamental life process. Do without it for a few days and the body will begin to fail. Continue the denial for several more days and total failure or irreparable damage will result. These things we know and accept and need no further convincing to firmly believe them.

I mentioned all this to make a point, which simply stated is drinking water is a natural procedure. We've been doing it since the beginning of life on earth. However, as we have evolved into the modern people we are, we have also evolved into people who do more eating than drinking. Further what little water we do drink is usually consumed at precisely the wrong time to be synergistic with our general digestive processes.

I have found over the years in which I have been implementing this regimen, that the timing that I use provides the best results and the least interference with easy digestion and proper absorption of the nutrients contained in the foods I normally eat. Let me quickly point out right here that there is nothing in my water intake regimen that precludes you from eating the foods that you're used to and normally consume. The key that will unlock the door to the slimmer person residing inside you is to drink the eight, (eight ounce glasses) of water per day as follows:

    . 2 glasses of water before breakfast

    . 2 glasses of water before lunch

    . 3 glasses of water before dinner

    . 1 glass of water before bedtime

It is important to note that I said "<u>before breakfast, before lunch and before dinner</u>". This I have found, by experience, is the key to the success of this plan.

My reasoning for the effectiveness of this plan is that by filling the stomach with water prior to eating cuts down on your desire to continue to fill the otherwise empty space in your belly. I have also found that during meals it is all right to drink a beverage, such as juice, diet soft drink, coffee, tea or even more water. However, I personally DO NOT consume any alcohol either with meals or at other times. Which brings me to the DO NOTS that my experience has taught me to observe.

DO NOT:

. Drink tap water. I drink only good bottled water or sparkling water

. Drink alcoholic beverages with your meal. I have found that alcoholic beverages have a tendency to increase your appetite.

. Eat between meals. Rather, do all your eating at meal times.

Again, I have found that I can eat anything I desire, even dessert during mealtime. Between meals, if you feel the need to put something in your stomach, have a glass of water instead. By the way, when drinking the water, I have found it's best to sip it and not chug-a-lug it. You'll find you'll actually begin to savor it as a boon companion while you go about the normal tasks that make up your everyday life.

NOTE: Many glasses, especially mugs are designed to hold twelve ounces normally contained in bottled and canned soft drinks. Make certain you use an eight-ounce glass. A simple check with a measuring cup is all that is required to be sure.   I mention this because of the experience of a friend of mine who decided to implement this regimen.   Several days went by before she discovered she was actually drinking fifty percent more water than I recommended. After that experience she found it easy to handle the eight-ounce glasses.

Chapter Three
Think Thin and Be Thin

Everything that happens inside our bodies does so in response to signals from our brain. Most of our bodily functions occur automatically with little conscious interference by the thinking part of our brain. However, the conscious part of the thinking part of our brain can and does influence bodily behavior in many ways. I have found that this is also true in its relationship to eating. While we're all victims of thoughtless behavior that we often unconsciously engage in, there are times when it would help us all to be more aware of this, often times, self-destructive practice.

As a case in point our appetite can subconsciously dictate our eating habits. When were hungry or otherwise stimulated to eat, we eat. However, this doesn't have to be left to a subconscious behavioral activity that snowballs to a point where our sizes snowball right along with it, but rather we can and should take

18

charge of the process. Thinking thin is the starting point of the process.

We have all heard enough about behavior modification to know that process has to begin in the brain. That is, in the conscious thinking part of the brain, and not the subconscious, non-thinking part of the brain, where most of our behavioral difficulties seem to reside. Therefore, a proper mental adjustment with a positive emphasis on being thin helps. Believe me I know, I think thin every day. There have been times when I have simply willed a few unwanted pounds away simply stressing in my mind the need to be rid of them. Of course, this required that I curtail my eating somewhat in addition to always following my daily regimen of water intake. But, the point I want to make is it has always been possible to do this with little or no discomfort, because I think thin and therefore I am thin.

So, I say to you, start by "thinking thin" and then proceed with determination to follow this simple regimen and you will not only achieve your desired weight goal, but you will be able to maintain it. The key understanding to put into your conscious mind is that by developing this simple easy to achieve habit, you will be able to continue to live your life as you currently do and not have to make any difficult adjustments.

Like all good things that last, my regimen will take a certain amount of time to take hold and begin to show its power to remove your undesired excess weight and then continue to control your weight for you. Here again, I stress the need to continue thinking thin by maintaining a positive attitude. This is so important because the brain plays funny tricks on us when we allow negative thoughts to dominate our thinking, like, "this doesn't work". Allow the seeds of doubt to plant themselves and the subconscious mind will be right back doing you down and dirty and guess what, you'll have still another weight loss program failure to contend with. "THINK POSITIVE"!

When you drink the recommended amount of water each day, the natural flushing mechanisms of the body's elimination system are allowed to do the job that nature intended. It's sort of like throwing the excess weight out with the wastewater. Further, a desirable side benefit of regularly cleansing the system is that a lot of toxins, and other bad things, the body has a tendency to store get washed away in the process. After all, the body is mostly water and represents extensive irrigation and filtration system. It was never intended to be a stagnant pool. Nature gave us water to drink to keep it from becoming one, so instead of a horse, lead yourself to water and for your own sake, drink it.

When you follow my regiment, you'll find that it is easy to implement no matter where you go, or what you're doing. Good bottled water is available nearly everywhere. So there is no need to lug large quantities with you if you go off for a few days or longer. Small bottles are also readily available to bring with you to work, school or anywhere you might be going for the day. To add a little zest to the game, use sparkling water along the way.

Chapter Four
EXERCISE

Exercise is a fundamentally important part of our existence. Like our predecessors we can or do get a lot of it during our normal course of living. Without going to any special pains to engage in a formal program there are many ways we can achieve continuous exercise throughout the course of our normal daily activities. All physical work is exercise in one form or another. Any activity, which requires body motion, is exercise if you think about it. Further, if you think some more about it that same working motion can be utilized as a more complete exercise simply by including some extra motions along with those required.

Look at it this way. As with problems, physical work can be viewed as opportunities to engage in additional exercise activities. Even when you are sitting down you can move your arms and legs; as a matter of fact it is good for you to do so. Many people I know who do sedentary work make a point to flex their muscles regularly, some have even told me that other people have commented about their "twitching". How about simply turning your head as far as it will go in each direction every so often and while you're at it looking off into the distance and bring your eyes to focus on what ever there is to be seen. Good for the neck muscles and good for the eyes.

Housework, the bane of most women's existence, is in reality still another opportunity to engage in regular exercise. Take your time and enjoy it. While pushing a vacuum cleaner back and forth swing your hips and step from side to side, all that motion is good for the "old bod" big time. Moving around the house is another way to exercise. Do it with deliberate movements, really get into it when you have to get up and go to the refrigerator or into the back bedroom to retrieve something you have left there. A walk out to the mailbox, is just that, a nice walk out in the fresh air. Take advantage of it with a light heart and good attitude and you may even find that you'll begin to take the long way there, just to extend the experience. Here again think positive, but most of all think and don't let your subconscious take over. It's your life, so live it in the best conscious way you can.

As your conscious mind begins to recapture its prerogatives and you find yourself thinking more about your activities, you will find many ways to amplify the ideas that I have set forth here. Exercising can be, and should be, a part of, and way of life. The idea that we need to block out special periods of time to accomplish it is to my way of thinking, utter nonsense. My own body tone and skin texture is proof of this and I haven't spent one minute inside a fitness studio (we use to call them gyms). I do have a bicycle, you know the kind we spend our childhood on, and I use that to run errands around the neighborhood and at times simply ride for the sheer enjoyment of it.

Now I have just about told my tale and here I would like to sum it all up.

1. Drink eight, eight ounce glasses of water each day.

2. Think thin, believe in yourself and you will achieve your desired weight level.

3. Take advantage of your natural exercise opportunities.

4. Greet everyday of your life with a positive attitude.

THINK THIN, BE HAPPY.

DO NOT GIVE UP.

YOU CAN DO IT!

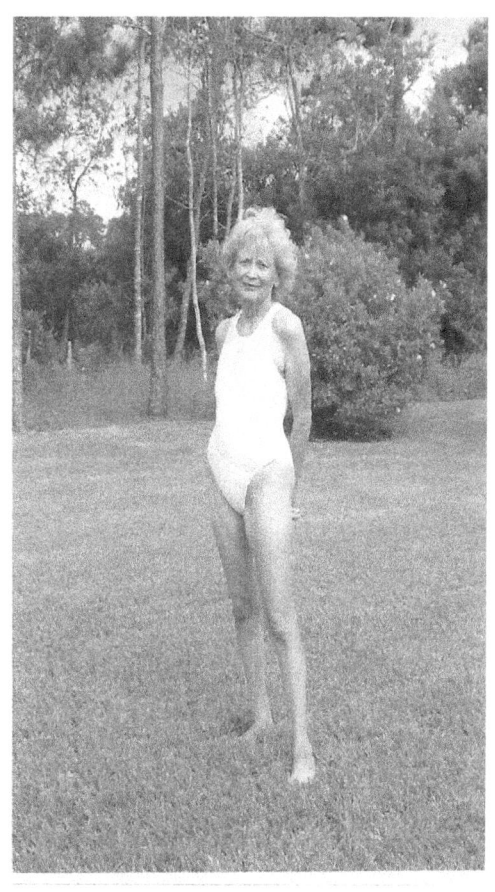

Picture Taken July 20, 2013
As of the original writing of this book in 2002, I was 72
years old. As you can see from the above picture, I still fit
in the same bathing suit and I am now **83 years old and
haven't changed that much. You can do it too!**